COMPLETE ARTHRITIS DIET COOKBOOK

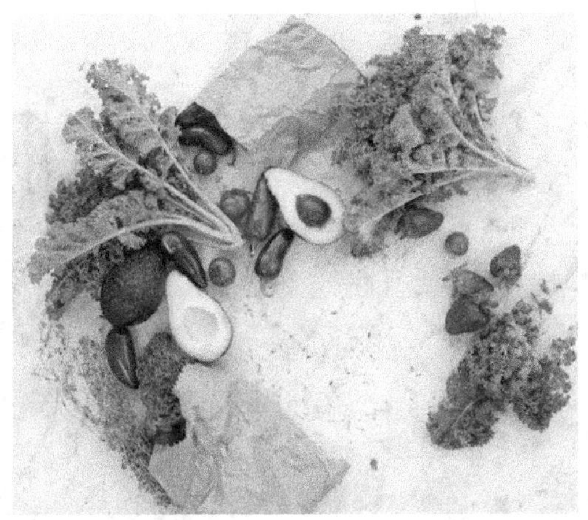

DR. JESSICA SMITH

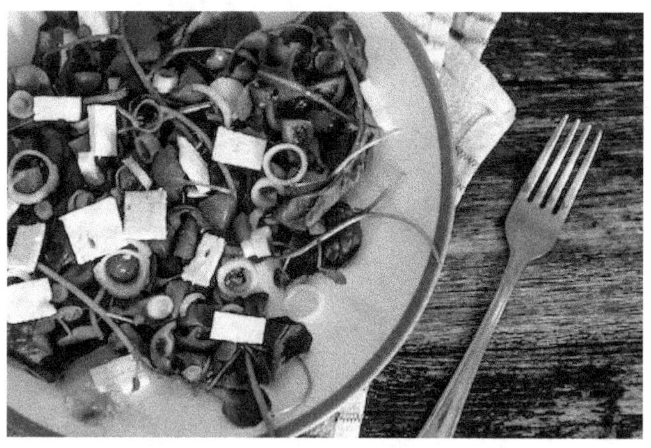

TABLE OF CONTENTS

CHAPTER ONE

Introduction Familiarization:

Start by reading the introduction section to understand the purpose of the cookbook and how it aligns with managing arthritis through diet.

Ingredient Exploration:

Take a thorough look at the ingredient lists provided for each recipe. Familiarize yourself with key elements, focusing on those known for anti-inflammatory and joint health benefits.

Understanding Dietary Guidelines:

Read the dietary guidelines and recommendations presented in the cookbook. This will help you understand the principles behind the recipes and how they contribute to arthritis management.

Meal Planning:

Use the cookbook as a tool for meal planning. Identify recipes that cater to your taste preferences and dietary needs while considering variety to ensure a well-balanced approach.

Educational Insights:

Pay attention to any educational insights or additional information offered with each recipe. This may include nutritional benefits, specific vitamins or minerals, and explanations about why certain ingredients are beneficial for arthritis.

Portion Control:

Be mindful of portion sizes. Controlling portions is crucial for managing weight, which is often associated with arthritis symptoms. The cookbook may provide guidance on appropriate serving sizes.

Variety Is Key:

Explore recipes across different categories—breakfast, lunch, dinner, snacks, and desserts. Incorporate a variety of foods to ensure a diverse range of nutrients beneficial for arthritis.

Experiment with Substitutions: Don't hesitate to experiment with ingredient substitutions to suit your taste and dietary preferences. Many recipes can be adapted based on personal needs.

Regular Reference:

Keep the cookbook handy for regular reference. This will make it easier to integrate arthritis-friendly recipes into your daily or weekly meal plans.

Feedback and Adaptation:

Finally, don't be afraid to provide feedback to yourself. Note which recipes you enjoy the most and any adjustments you make. This cookbook is a tool for your journey, and adapting it to your needs is encouraged.

Understanding Complete Arthritis Diet

Understanding the Complete Arthritis Diet involves grasping the intricate connection between nutrition and the management of arthritis symptoms.

This comprehensive approach to dietary choices aims to alleviates inflammation, reduce joint pain, and enhance overall joint health. The foundation lies in selecting foods that possess anti-inflammatory properties, such as omega-3 fatty acids, antioxidants, and specific vitamins and minerals.

The Complete Arthritis Diet emphasizes the consumption of whole, nutrient-dense foods, including fruits, vegetables, lean proteins, and healthy fats.

It discourages the intake of processed foods, sugars, and saturated fats, which can exacerbate inflammation and contribute to weight gain – a factor closely linked to arthritis discomfort.

In addition to individual recipes, this diet plan often provides valuable insights into the science behind the chosen ingredients.

Understanding the benefits of foods like fatty fish, leafy greens, and nuts empowers individuals to make informed choices that positively impact their joint health.

Moreover, the diet may encourage maintaining a healthy weight, as excess body weight places additional stress on joints.

By adhering to the principles outlined in the Complete Arthritis Diet, individuals can cultivate habits that contribute to overall well-being and potentially experience a reduction in arthritis-related symptoms.

This dietary approach transcends mere eating; it embodies a lifestyle that nurtures joint health and fosters a sense of empowerment in managing arthritis.

Principles of Complete Arthritis Diet

The principles of the Complete Arthritis Diet revolve around harnessing the healing power of nutrition to manage arthritis symptoms effectively.

These guiding principles encompass a holistic approach that considers the inflammatory nature of arthritis and the role of certain foods in either exacerbating or alleviating joint discomfort.

Anti-Inflammatory Foods: The diet prioritizes foods with proven anti-inflammatory properties, such as fatty fish rich in omega-3 fatty acids, colorful fruits and vegetables teeming with antioxidants, and nuts and seeds containing essential nutrients that support joint health.

Balanced Nutrition: A key principle is maintaining a well-balanced diet that provides a spectrum of essential nutrients. This includes a focus on lean proteins for muscle support, whole grains for sustained energy, and a variety of vitamins and minerals crucial for overall health.

Omega-3 Fatty Acids: Incorporating sources of omega-3 fatty acids, such as salmon, flaxseeds, and walnuts, is a cornerstone. These fats have been linked to reduced inflammation and can play a vital role in managing arthritis symptoms.

Limiting Inflammatory Culprits: Conversely, the diet discourages the consumption of foods known to promote inflammation, such as processed foods, sugary treats, and saturated fats found in certain meats and fried items.

Hydration: Ensuring adequate hydration is vital. Water is essential for joint lubrication and overall bodily functions, contributing to the overall health of individuals managing arthritis.

Mindful Eating: The principles encourage mindful eating practices, emphasizing the importance of savoring meals, recognizing hunger and fullness cues, and cultivating a positive relationship with food.

Weight Management: Maintaining a healthy weight is integral, as excess weight places additional stress on joints. The diet supports weight management through nutrient-dense, lower-calorie options.

The benefits of the Complete Arthritis Diet extend far beyond the realm of mere nutrition, offering a holistic approach that positively impacts joint health and overall well-being. Embracing this dietary strategy can bring about a range of advantages for individuals grappling with arthritis symptoms.

Reduced Inflammation: A cornerstone benefit is the potential to reduce inflammation, a primary driver of arthritis discomfort. The diet's emphasis on anti-inflammatory foods, such as fatty fish, leafy greens, and berries, can contribute to calming inflammatory responses within the body.

Joint Pain Relief: By incorporating foods rich in omega-3 fatty acids, like salmon and chia seeds, individuals may experience alleviation of joint pain. Omega-3s have been shown to have anti-inflammatory and analgesic properties, offering relief from arthritis-related discomfort.

Improved Joint Mobility: The Complete Arthritis Diet promotes the consumption of nutrient-dense foods that support joint health. Essential nutrients, including vitamins

C and D, as well as minerals like calcium, contribute to improved joint mobility and flexibility.

Weight Management: As the diet encourages a focus on whole, nutrient-dense foods and discourages inflammatory culprits like processed items and sugary treats, it aids in weight management. Maintaining a healthy weight is crucial for individuals with arthritis, as excess weight can exacerbate joint pain.

Enhanced Overall Well-being: Beyond arthritis-specific benefits, the diet's emphasis on balanced nutrition contributes to overall health. Nutrient-rich foods support immune function, boost energy levels, and foster a sense of well-being.

Potential Disease Modifying Effects: Some elements of the diet, particularly those rich in antioxidants and anti-inflammatory compounds, may have disease-modifying effects. While not a cure, adopting this dietary approach can positively impact the progression of arthritis.

Empowerment and Control: Perhaps one of the most significant benefits is the sense of empowerment and control that individuals gain over their health.

The Complete Arthritis Diet becomes a tool for self-care, fostering a proactive approach to managing arthritis symptoms through mindful and intentional dietary choices.

Tips for Complete Arthritis Diet

Navigating the Complete Arthritis Diet successfully involves incorporating mindful habits and making informed choices. Here are essential tips to enhance your experience with this dietary approach:

Consult with a Healthcare Professional: Before making significant changes to your diet, consult with a healthcare professional or a registered dietitian. They can provide personalized guidance based on your specific health needs and conditions.

Gradual Changes: Introduce dietary changes gradually. This allows your body to adjust and helps you identify how different foods impact your arthritis symptoms.

Keep a Food Journal: Maintain a food journal to track your diet and note any changes in arthritis symptoms. This can be a valuable tool for identifying trigger foods or recognizing patterns that affect your joint health.

Embrace Variety: Include a diverse range of fruits, vegetables, lean proteins, and whole grains in your diet. Variety ensures you receive a broad spectrum of nutrients beneficial for joint health.

Mindful Eating: Practice mindful eating by savoring each bite, paying attention to hunger and fullness cues, and cultivating a positive relationship with food. This approach can enhance your overall dining experience.

Hydration Matters: Stay adequately hydrated. Water is essential for joint lubrication and overall bodily functions. Limiting sugary and caffeinated beverages is advisable.

Consider Supplements: While obtaining nutrients from whole foods is optimal, some individuals may require supplements. Discuss potential supplementation with your healthcare provider to ensure you meet your nutritional needs.

Experiment with Cooking Techniques: Explore different cooking techniques. Steaming, baking, and grilling are healthier alternatives to frying. These methods retain more nutrients and contribute to joint-friendly meals.

Read Labels: Develop the habit of reading food labels. Look for hidden sugars, artificial additives, and excessive sodium, as these can contribute to inflammation and joint discomfort.

Be Flexible: Recognize that dietary needs may vary. Be flexible and adjust your diet based on your body's responses. Listen to how your joints react to certain foods and make modifications accordingly.

Guidelines for Complete Arthritis Diet

Guidelines for the Complete Arthritis Diet serve as a roadmap for individuals seeking to manage arthritis symptoms through thoughtful dietary choices.

These guidelines encompass a holistic approach, emphasizing not just what to eat but also fostering a lifestyle that supports joint health and overall well-being.

Focus on Anti-Inflammatory Foods: Prioritize foods known for their anti-inflammatory properties, such as fatty fish (salmon, mackerel), leafy greens, berries, nuts, and seeds. These can help mitigate inflammation and alleviate joint pain.

Incorporate Omega-3 Fatty Acids: Embrace sources of omega-3 fatty acids, such as flaxseeds, chia seeds, walnuts, and fatty fish. These essential fats have demonstrated anti-inflammatory effects and are crucial for joint health.

Colorful Plate: Aim for a colorful plate by including a variety of fruits and vegetables. Vibrant colors often indicate a rich concentration of antioxidants, which can combat oxidative stress and support joint health.

Lean Proteins: Choose lean protein sources like poultry, fish, beans, and legumes. Protein is essential for muscle support and overall joint function.

Whole Grains: Opt for whole grains such as brown rice, quinoa, and oats. These provide fiber and essential nutrients without the inflammatory effects associated with refined grains.

Limit Inflammatory Culprits: Reduce the intake of foods that can trigger inflammation, including processed foods, sugary treats, and saturated fats found in certain meats and fried items.

Stay Hydrated: Hydration is crucial for joint lubrication. Consume an adequate amount of water throughout the day and limit the consumption of sugary and caffeinated beverages.

Moderate Portion Sizes: Practice portion control to maintain a healthy weight. Excess weight can exacerbate arthritis symptoms, particularly in weight-bearing joints.

Mindful Eating: Engage in mindful eating practices. Pay attention to hunger and fullness cues, savor each bite, and cultivate a positive relationship with food.

Consult Healthcare Professionals: Before making significant changes to your diet, consult with healthcare professionals or a registered dietitian. They can provide personalized guidance based on your health status and dietary needs.

Causes of Arthritis

Arthritis, a term encompassing over 100 different conditions affecting the joints, is characterized by inflammation, pain, and stiffness.

The causes of arthritis are diverse and multifaceted, often involving a combination of genetic, environmental, and lifestyle factors.

Genetic Predisposition: Family history plays a significant role in certain types of arthritis. Genetic factors can increase susceptibility to conditions like rheumatoid arthritis, osteoarthritis, and ankylosing spondylitis.

Age: The risk of developing arthritis tends to increase with age. Osteoarthritis, the most common form, is often associated with the wear and tear of joints over time.

Joint Injuries: Trauma or injuries to the joints, such as fractures or dislocations, can contribute to the development of arthritis. Injured joints may be more prone to inflammation and damage.

Autoimmune Disorders: Conditions like rheumatoid arthritis and lupus involve the immune system mistakenly attacking the body's own tissues, leading to joint inflammation and damage.

Infections: Some infections, particularly those affecting the joints, can trigger certain types of arthritis. Bacterial, viral, or fungal infections may contribute to the development of reactive arthritis.

Metabolic Factors: Conditions like gout are associated with metabolic factors. Excessive uric acid in the blood can crystallize and deposit in joints, causing inflammation and pain.

Gender and Hormones: Women are more commonly affected by certain types of arthritis, such as rheumatoid arthritis. Hormonal factors may contribute to this gender disparity.

Obesity: Excess weight places additional stress on weight-bearing joints, contributing to the development and progression of osteoarthritis. Obesity is a known risk factor for arthritis.

Environmental Factors: Environmental influences, such as exposure to cigarette smoke, air pollution, and occupational hazards, may contribute to the development of certain types of arthritis.

Understanding the various causes of arthritis is crucial for effective management and prevention strategies.

While some factors are beyond individual control, adopting a healthy lifestyle, maintaining a balanced diet, and seeking early medical intervention can play pivotal roles in mitigating the impact of arthritis.

Arthritis encompasses a diverse array of conditions, each characterized by inflammation of the joints, leading to pain, stiffness, and reduced mobility.

Here are some prominent types of arthritis:

Osteoarthritis (OA): The most common type, OA is associated with the wear and tear of joints over time. It typically affects weight-bearing joints like the knees, hips, and spine, causing cartilage breakdown and joint pain.

Rheumatoid Arthritis (RA): An autoimmune disorder where the immune system mistakenly attacks the synovium, the lining of the membranes surrounding the joints. This chronic inflammation can lead to joint deformities and damage.

Psoriatic Arthritis (PsA): Occurring in individuals with psoriasis, PsA affects both the skin and joints. It can cause joint pain, swelling, and skin lesions.

Ankylosing Spondylitis (AS): Primarily affecting the spine, AS causes inflammation in the vertebrae, leading to stiffness and reduced flexibility. It may also affect other joints and organs.

Gout: Caused by the accumulation of uric acid crystals in the joints, gout typically affects the big toe. It leads to sudden and severe pain, inflammation, and redness.

Lupus Arthritis: A component of systemic lupus erythematosus (SLE), lupus arthritis involves joint pain, stiffness, and swelling as part of the autoimmune response.

Juvenile Idiopathic Arthritis (JIA): This refers to a group of arthritis conditions that occur in children under the age of 16, characterized by joint inflammation lasting for at least six weeks.

Infectious Arthritis: Caused by bacteria, viruses, or fungi entering the joint, infectious arthritis leads to inflammation. Prompt treatment is essential to prevent joint damage.

Reactive Arthritis: Arising as a response to an infection elsewhere in the body, reactive arthritis typically affects the joints, eyes, and urinary tract.

Symptoms of arthritis can vary widely depending on the specific type of arthritis, but they generally revolve around joint inflammation, pain, stiffness, and impaired mobility. Here are common symptoms associated with arthritis:

Joint Pain: Persistent or recurring pain in one or more joints is a hallmark symptom of arthritis. The intensity and location of pain can vary based on the type of arthritis.

Joint Swelling: Inflammation within the joints often leads to swelling, causing the affected areas to appear larger, warmer, and tender to the touch.

Stiffness: Arthritis-related stiffness is usually most pronounced in the morning or after periods of inactivity. It can limit joint movement and gradually improve with gentle activity.

Redness and Warmth: Inflamed joints may exhibit redness and warmth due to increased blood flow to the affected area.

Reduced Range of Motion: Arthritis can restrict the normal range of motion in affected joints, making it challenging to perform daily activities that involve movement.

Fatigue: Chronic pain and inflammation can contribute to fatigue, affecting overall energy levels and well-being.

Joint Deformities: In some types of arthritis, prolonged inflammation can lead to joint deformities, particularly in conditions like rheumatoid arthritis.

Fever and General Malaise: Systemic symptoms, including fever and a general feeling of unwellness, can accompany certain types of inflammatory arthritis.

Skin Changes: Conditions like psoriatic arthritis may involve skin changes, including psoriasis lesions on the skin.

Eye Issues: Inflammatory arthritis types like ankylosing spondylitis or reactive arthritis may cause eye inflammation, leading to redness and pain.

It's essential to note that arthritis symptoms can fluctuate, with periods of exacerbation (flares) and improvement.

Early diagnosis and appropriate management are crucial for effectively addressing symptoms and preventing long-term joint damage.

Individuals experiencing persistent joint-related symptoms should seek medical evaluation for an accurate diagnosis and tailored treatment plan.

Risk Factor of Arthritis

Arthritis is influenced by a combination of genetic, environmental, and lifestyle factors. Several risk factors contribute to the development and progression of various types of arthritis:

Age: The risk of arthritis increases with age. Osteoarthritis, the most common type, is often associated with the natural wear and tear of joints over time.

Gender: Certain types of arthritis, such as rheumatoid arthritis, are more prevalent in women. However, gout is more common in men.

Family History: Genetic factors play a significant role. Individuals with a family history of arthritis, particularly rheumatoid arthritis or ankylosing spondylitis, may have an increased risk.

Previous Joint Injuries: Trauma, joint injuries, or surgeries can elevate the risk of developing arthritis. Injuries may lead to joint instability and increased susceptibility to inflammation.

Obesity: Excess body weight places additional stress on joints, particularly in weight-bearing areas like the knees and hips. This can contribute to the development and progression of arthritis, especially osteoarthritis.

Infections: Certain infections, such as those affecting the joints or causing inflammatory responses, can increase the risk of developing specific types of arthritis, like reactive arthritis.

Occupational Hazards: Occupations involving repetitive joint movements, heavy lifting, or exposure to joint-damaging substances may contribute to arthritis development.

Smoking: Smoking has been linked to an increased risk of developing rheumatoid arthritis. It may also exacerbate symptoms in individuals already diagnosed with arthritis.

Hormones: Hormonal factors, particularly in women, may influence the risk of developing arthritis. Hormonal changes can affect the immune system and contribute to joint inflammation.

Chronic Diseases: Individuals with certain chronic conditions, such as diabetes, may have an elevated risk of developing specific types of arthritis.

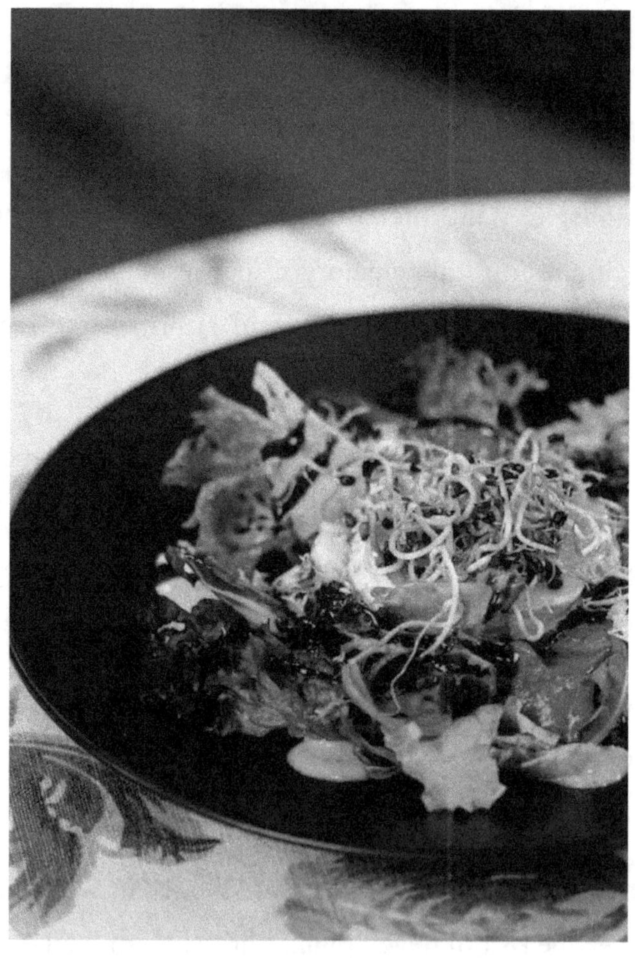

CHAPTER TWO

1: Berry-Oat Breakfast Bowl

Ingredients:

- 1/2 cup rolled oats
- 1 cup mixed berries (blueberries, strawberries, raspberries)
- 1 tablespoon chia seeds
- 1 tablespoon chopped nuts (almonds, walnuts)
- 1 teaspoon honey
- 1 cup almond milk

Instructions:

- Combine rolled oats and almond milk in a bowl.
- Add mixed berries, chia seeds, and chopped nuts.
- Drizzle honey on top.
- Mix well and let it sit in the refrigerator overnight.
- In the morning, stir the mixture and enjoy this nutrient-packed bowl.

Health Benefits:

> Oats provide fiber and antioxidants.

> Berries offer anti-inflammatory compounds.

> Chia seeds and nuts contribute omega-3 fatty acids.

Preparation Time: 10 minutes (plus overnight soaking)

2: Avocado Toast with Poached Egg

Ingredients:

> 1 slice whole-grain bread

> 1/2 ripe avocado

> 1 poached egg

> Salt and pepper to taste

> Optional: sprinkle of turmeric

Instructions:

> Toast the whole-grain bread.

> Mash the ripe avocado and spread it on the toast.

> Place the poached egg on top.

> Season with salt, pepper, and turmeric if desired.

Health Benefits:

> Whole-grain bread provides fiber.

- ➤ Avocado offers healthy fats and anti-inflammatory properties.
- ➤ Eggs are a good source of protein.

Preparation Time: 15 minutes

3: Turmeric Smoothie

Ingredients:

- ➤ 1 cup coconut milk
- ➤ 1/2 frozen banana
- ➤ 1/2 cup pineapple chunks
- ➤ 1/2 teaspoon turmeric powder
- ➤ 1/2 teaspoon ginger powder
- ➤ 1 tablespoon chia seeds

Instructions:

- ➤ Blend coconut milk, frozen banana, pineapple, turmeric, and ginger until smooth.
- ➤ Pour into a glass and stir in chia seeds.

Health Benefits:

- ➤ Turmeric and ginger have anti-inflammatory properties.
- ➤ Chia seeds provide omega-3 fatty acids.

Preparation Time: 5 minutes

4: Spinach and Feta Omelette

Ingredients:

- 2 eggs, beaten
- Handful of fresh spinach
- 2 tablespoons crumbled feta cheese
- 1/4 red bell pepper, diced
- Salt and pepper to taste

Instructions:

- Sauté spinach and bell pepper in a pan until wilted.
- Pour beaten eggs over the vegetables.
- Sprinkle feta cheese on top.
- Cook until the eggs are set, then fold the omelette.

Health Benefits:

- Spinach provides iron and vitamins.
- Feta adds calcium and protein.

Preparation Time: 10 minutes

Ingredients:

- 1/2 cup cooked quinoa
- 1/2 cup Greek yogurt
- 1/4 cup mixed berries
- 1 tablespoon honey
- 1 tablespoon chopped almonds

Instructions:

- Layer cooked quinoa, Greek yogurt, and mixed berries in a bowl.
- Drizzle with honey and sprinkle chopped almonds on top.

Health Benefits:

- Quinoa offers protein and fiber.
- Greek yogurt provides probiotics and calcium.
- Berries contribute antioxidants.

Preparation Time: 15 minutes

6: Salmon and Avocado Breakfast Wrap

Ingredients:

- 1 whole-grain tortilla
- 2 oz smoked salmon
- 1/2 ripe avocado, sliced
- 1 tablespoon cream cheese
- Fresh dill for garnish

Instructions:

- Spread cream cheese on the tortilla.
- Layer smoked salmon and sliced avocado.
- Garnish with fresh dill.
- Roll into a wrap and slice.

Health Benefits:

- Salmon provides omega-3 fatty acids.
- Avocado offers healthy fats and anti-inflammatory properties.

Preparation Time: 10 minutes

Ingredients:

- 2 tablespoons chia seeds
- 1/2 cup almond milk
- 1/4 cup fresh blueberries
- 1 tablespoon almond butter
- 1 teaspoon honey

Instructions:

- Mix chia seeds with almond milk and let it sit for 15 minutes.
- Layer chia pudding with fresh blueberries.
- Drizzle almond butter and honey on top.

Health Benefits:

- Chia seeds provide omega-3 fatty acids and fiber.
- Blueberries offer antioxidants.

Preparation Time: 20 minutes (including soaking time)

8: Sweet Potato and Kale Hash

Ingredients:

- 1 medium sweet potato, grated

- ➢ 1 cup kale, chopped

- ➢ 1/4 red onion, finely chopped

- ➢ 1 clove garlic, minced

- ➢ 2 eggs

- ➢ Salt and pepper to taste

Instructions:

- ➢ Sauté sweet potato, kale, red onion, and garlic in a pan until tender.

- ➢ Make two wells in the hash and crack eggs into them.

- ➢ Cover and cook until eggs are done to your liking.

Health Benefits:

- ➢ Sweet potatoes offer vitamins and antioxidants.

- ➢ Kale provides anti-inflammatory compounds.

Preparation Time: 15 minutes

9: Quinoa and Vegetable Breakfast Skillet

Ingredients:

- ➢ 1 cup cooked quinoa

- ➢ 1/2 cup cherry tomatoes, halved

- ➢ 1/4 cup bell peppers, diced

- ➢ 2 green onions, chopped

- ➤ 1 tablespoon olive oil
- ➤ 2 eggs

Instructions:

- ➤ Sauté cherry tomatoes, bell peppers, and green onions in olive oil.
- ➤ Add cooked quinoa and stir.
- ➤ Make two wells and crack eggs into them.
- ➤ Cover and cook until eggs are done.

Health Benefits:

- ➤ Quinoa provides protein and fiber.
- ➤ Vegetables offer vitamins and antioxidants.

Preparation Time: 15 minutes

10: Banana Walnut Overnight Oats

Ingredients:

- ➤ 1/2 cup rolled oats
- ➤ 1/2 cup almond milk
- ➤ 1/2 ripe banana, mashed
- ➤ 1 tablespoon chopped walnuts
- ➤ 1 teaspoon maple syrup

Instructions:

> ➢ Mix rolled oats, almond milk, mashed banana, and chopped walnuts in a jar.
> ➢ Refrigerate overnight.
> ➢ Drizzle with maple syrup before serving.

Health Benefits:

> ➢ Oats provide fiber and antioxidants.
> ➢ Bananas offer potassium and natural sweetness.
> ➢ Walnuts contribute omega-3 fatty acids.

Preparation Time: 5 minutes (plus overnight soaking)

Lunch Recipes for Arthritis

1: Quinoa and Chickpea Salad

Ingredients:

> ➢ 1 cup cooked quinoa
> ➢ 1 can (15 oz) chickpeas, drained and rinsed
> ➢ 1 cucumber, diced
> ➢ 1 cup cherry tomatoes, halved
> ➢ 1/4 cup red onion, finely chopped
> ➢ Feta cheese crumbles (optional)
> ➢ Fresh parsley, chopped

➤ Olive oil and lemon dressing

Instructions:

➤ In a large bowl, combine quinoa, chickpeas, cucumber, cherry tomatoes, and red onion.

➤ Toss with olive oil and lemon dressing.

➤ Top with feta cheese crumbles and fresh parsley.

Health Benefits:

➤ Quinoa provides protein and fiber.

➤ Chickpeas offer protein and anti-inflammatory properties.

Preparation Time: 20 minutes

2: Salmon and Avocado Salad

Ingredients:

➤ 6 oz grilled salmon, flaked

➤ Mixed salad greens

➤ 1 avocado, sliced

➤ 1/4 cup cherry tomatoes, halved

➤ 1/4 cup cucumber, sliced

➤ Balsamic vinaigrette dressing

Instructions:

> Arrange salad greens on a plate.
> Top with grilled salmon, avocado slices, cherry tomatoes, and cucumber.
> Drizzle with balsamic vinaigrette dressing.

Health Benefits:

> Salmon provides omega-3 fatty acids.
> Avocado offers healthy fats and anti-inflammatory properties.

Preparation Time: 15 minutes

3: Lentil and Vegetable Soup

Ingredients:

> 1 cup green lentils, rinsed
> 1 onion, diced
> 2 carrots, diced
> 2 celery stalks, diced
> 3 cloves garlic, minced
> 6 cups vegetable broth
> 1 teaspoon cumin
> 1 teaspoon turmeric

➢ Salt and pepper to taste

Instructions:

➢ In a large pot, sauté onion, carrots, celery, and garlic until softened.
➢ Add lentils, vegetable broth, cumin, turmeric, salt, and pepper.
➢ Simmer until lentils are tender.

Health Benefits:

➢ Lentils provide protein and fiber.
➢ Turmeric and cumin offer anti-inflammatory properties.

Preparation Time: 30 minutes

4: Turkey and Quinoa Stuffed Peppers

Ingredients:

➢ 4 bell peppers, halved and seeds removed
➢ 1 cup cooked quinoa
➢ 1 lb ground turkey
➢ 1 onion, diced
➢ 1 can (15 oz) diced tomatoes
➢ 1 teaspoon Italian seasoning

> Salt and pepper to taste

Instructions:

> Preheat the oven to 375°F (190°C).
> In a skillet, cook ground turkey and onions until browned.
> Add cooked quinoa, diced tomatoes, Italian seasoning, salt, and pepper.
> Stuff bell peppers with the turkey and quinoa mixture.
> Bake for 25-30 minutes until peppers are tender.

Health Benefits:

> Quinoa provides protein and fiber.
> Turkey offers lean protein.

Preparation Time: 45 minutes

5: Spinach and Mushroom Quiche

Ingredients:

> 1 whole-grain pie crust
> 1 cup fresh spinach, chopped
> 1 cup mushrooms, sliced
> 4 eggs

> 1 cup milk (dairy or plant-based)

> 1/2 cup feta cheese (optional)

> Salt and pepper to taste

Instructions:

> Preheat the oven to 375°F (190°C).

> Sauté spinach and mushrooms until wilted.

> In a bowl, whisk together eggs, milk, feta cheese, salt, and pepper.

> Pour the egg mixture into the pie crust.

> Add the sautéed spinach and mushrooms.

> Bake for 35-40 minutes until the quiche is set.

Health Benefits:

> Spinach provides iron and vitamins.

> Mushrooms offer antioxidants.

Preparation Time: 50 minutes

6: Mediterranean Chickpea Salad Wrap

Ingredients:

> 1 can (15 oz) chickpeas, drained and rinsed

> 1 cup cherry tomatoes, halved

> 1 cucumber, diced

- ➤ 1/4 cup red onion, finely chopped
- ➤ Kalamata olives, sliced
- ➤ Feta cheese crumbles
- ➤ Whole-grain wraps

Instructions:

- ➤ In a bowl, combine chickpeas, cherry tomatoes, cucumber, red onion, and olives.
- ➤ Spoon the mixture onto whole-grain wraps.
- ➤ Top with feta cheese crumbles.
- ➤ Roll into wraps and serve.

Health Benefits:

- ➤ Chickpeas provide protein and anti-inflammatory properties.
- ➤ Tomatoes and cucumbers offer vitamins and antioxidants.

Preparation Time: 15 minutes

7: Cauliflower Fried Rice with Shrimp

Ingredients:

- ➤ 2 cups cauliflower rice
- ➤ 1/2 lb shrimp, peeled and deveined

- ➢ 1 cup mixed vegetables (peas, carrots, corn)
- ➢ 2 eggs, beaten
- ➢ 2 tablespoons soy sauce (low sodium)
- ➢ 1 tablespoon sesame oil
- ➢ Green onions for garnish

Instructions:

- ➢ In a pan, cook shrimp until pink.
- ➢ Add mixed vegetables and cauliflower rice.
- ➢ Push ingredients to one side and scramble eggs on the other side.
- ➢ Mix everything together, add soy sauce and sesame oil.
- ➢ Garnish with chopped green onions.

Health Benefits:

- ➢ Cauliflower provides a low-carb alternative to rice.
- ➢ Shrimp offers lean protein.

Preparation Time: 20 minutes

8: Greek Chicken Salad

Ingredients:

- ➢ 1 lb chicken breasts, grilled and sliced

- Mixed salad greens
- Cherry tomatoes, halved
- Cucumber, sliced
- Red onion, thinly sliced
- Feta cheese crumbles
- Kalamata olives
- Greek dressing

Instructions:

- Arrange salad greens on a plate.
- Top with grilled chicken, cherry tomatoes, cucumber, red onion, feta cheese, and olives.
- Drizzle with Greek dressing.

Health Benefits:

- Chicken provides lean protein.
- Feta and olives offer healthy fats and antioxidants.

Preparation Time: 20 minutes

9: Sweet Potato and Black Bean Quesadillas

Ingredients:

- 2 whole-grain tortillas
- 1 cup sweet potatoes, roasted and mashed

- ➢ 1/2 cup black beans, cooked
- ➢ 1/4 cup red onion, diced
- ➢ 1/2 cup shredded cheese (cheddar or Mexican blend)
- ➢ Guacamole for serving

Instructions:

- ➢ Spread mashed sweet potatoes on one side of each tortilla.
- ➢ Top one tortilla with black beans, red onion, and shredded cheese.
- ➢ Place the other tortilla on top.
- ➢ Cook in a skillet until the cheese melts.
- ➢ Slice into wedges and serve with guacamole.

Health Benefits:

- ➢ Sweet potatoes offer vitamins and fiber.
- ➢ Black beans provide protein and fiber.

Preparation Time: 25 minutes

10: Asian-Inspired Tofu Stir-Fry

Ingredients:

- ➢ 1 block firm tofu, pressed and cubed

- ➤ Mixed stir-fry vegetables (broccoli, bell peppers, snap peas)
- ➤ 2 tablespoons soy sauce (low sodium)
- ➤ 1 tablespoon hoisin sauce
- ➤ 1 teaspoon sesame oil
- ➤ 1 tablespoon vegetable oil
- ➤ Brown rice for serving

Instructions:

- ➤ In a pan, heat vegetable oil and stir-fry tofu until golden.
- ➤ Add mixed vegetables and continue to stir-fry.
- ➤ Pour in soy sauce, hoisin sauce, and sesame oil.
- ➤ Serve over brown rice.

Health Benefits:

- ➤ Tofu provides plant-based protein.
- ➤ Mixed vegetables offer vitamins and antioxidants.

Preparation Time: 30 minutes

1: Baked Lemon Herb Salmon

Ingredients:

- 4 salmon fillets
- 2 tablespoons olive oil
- 2 tablespoons fresh lemon juice
- 1 teaspoon dried thyme
- 1 teaspoon dried rosemary
- Salt and pepper to taste
- Lemon slices for garnish

Instructions:

- Preheat the oven to 375°F (190°C).
- Place salmon fillets on a baking sheet.
- Mix olive oil, lemon juice, thyme, rosemary, salt, and pepper in a bowl.
- Brush the salmon with the mixture.
- Bake for 15-20 minutes or until the salmon is cooked through.
- Garnish with lemon slices before serving.

Health Benefits:

> Salmon provides omega-3 fatty acids.
> Lemon and herbs offer anti-inflammatory properties.

Preparation Time: 25 minutes

2: Quinoa and Vegetable Stuffed Bell Peppers

Ingredients:

> 4 bell peppers, halved and seeds removed
> 1 cup cooked quinoa
> 1 can (15 oz) black beans, drained and rinsed
> 1 cup corn kernels
> 1 cup cherry tomatoes, diced
> 1/2 cup red onion, finely chopped
> 1 teaspoon cumin
> 1 teaspoon chili powder
> Shredded cheese for topping (optional)

Instructions:

> Preheat the oven to 375°F (190°C).
> In a bowl, mix quinoa, black beans, corn, cherry tomatoes, red onion, cumin, and chili powder.
> Stuff bell peppers with the quinoa mixture.

- ➢ Top with shredded cheese if desired.

- ➢ Bake for 25-30 minutes until peppers are tender.

Health Benefits:

- ➢ Quinoa provides protein and fiber.

- ➢ Black beans offer protein and anti-inflammatory properties.

Preparation Time: 40 minutes

3: Chicken and Broccoli Stir-Fry

Ingredients:

- ➢ 1 lb boneless, skinless chicken breasts, sliced

- ➢ 2 cups broccoli florets

- ➢ 1 bell pepper, sliced

- ➢ 2 tablespoons soy sauce (low sodium)

- ➢ 1 tablespoon honey

- ➢ 1 tablespoon sesame oil

- ➢ 1 tablespoon olive oil

- ➢ 2 cloves garlic, minced

- ➢ Brown rice for serving

Instructions:

> In a wok or skillet, heat olive oil and cook chicken until browned.
> Add broccoli, bell pepper, and garlic. Stir-fry until vegetables are tender-crisp.
> In a small bowl, mix soy sauce, honey, and sesame oil. Pour over the chicken and vegetables.
> Serve over brown rice.

Health Benefits:

> Chicken provides lean protein.
> Broccoli offers vitamins and anti-inflammatory compounds.

Preparation Time: 30 minutes

4: Lentil and Vegetable Curry

Ingredients:

> 1 cup dry lentils, rinsed
> 1 onion, diced
> 2 carrots, sliced
> 2 potatoes, diced
> 1 can (15 oz) diced tomatoes

- ➢ 1 can (15 oz) coconut milk
- ➢ 2 tablespoons curry powder
- ➢ 1 teaspoon turmeric
- ➢ Salt and pepper to taste
- ➢ Fresh cilantro for garnish
- ➢ Basmati rice for serving

Instructions:

- ➢ In a large pot, combine lentils, onion, carrots, potatoes, diced tomatoes, coconut milk, curry powder, turmeric, salt, and pepper.
- ➢ Bring to a boil, then simmer until lentils and vegetables are tender.
- ➢ Serve over basmati rice and garnish with fresh cilantro.

Health Benefits:

- ➢ Lentils provide protein and fiber.
- ➢ Turmeric offers anti-inflammatory properties.

Preparation Time: 40 minutes

5: Turkey and Sweet Potato Skillet

Ingredients:

- ➢ 1 lb ground turkey
- ➢ 2 sweet potatoes, peeled and diced
- ➢ 1 bell pepper, diced
- ➢ 1 zucchini, sliced
- ➢ 2 cloves garlic, minced
- ➢ 1 teaspoon cumin
- ➢ 1 teaspoon paprika
- ➢ Salt and pepper to taste
- ➢ Fresh parsley for garnish

Instructions:

- ➢ In a large skillet, cook ground turkey until browned.
- ➢ Add sweet potatoes, bell pepper, zucchini, garlic, cumin, paprika, salt, and pepper.
- ➢ Cover and cook until sweet potatoes are tender.
- ➢ Garnish with fresh parsley before serving.

Health Benefits:

- ➢ Turkey provides lean protein.
- ➢ Sweet potatoes offer vitamins and antioxidants.

Preparation Time: 35 minutes

6: Mediterranean Quinoa Bowl

Ingredients:

- 1 cup cooked quinoa
- 1 cup cherry tomatoes, halved
- 1 cucumber, diced
- 1/2 cup Kalamata olives, sliced
- 1/2 cup feta cheese, crumbled
- Red onion, thinly sliced
- Fresh oregano for garnish
- Greek dressing

Instructions:

- In a bowl, combine quinoa, cherry tomatoes, cucumber, olives, feta cheese, and red onion.
- Drizzle with Greek dressing and toss gently.
- Garnish with fresh oregano before serving.

Health Benefits:

- Quinoa provides protein and fiber.
- Kalamata olives and feta offer healthy fats and antioxidants.

Preparation Time: 20 minutes

7: Chickpea and Vegetable Skewers

Ingredients:

> 1 can (15 oz) chickpeas, drained and rinsed

> Cherry tomatoes

> Zucchini, sliced

> Bell peppers, cut into chunks

> Red onion, cut into wedges

> Olive oil and lemon marinade

> Fresh herbs (rosemary, thyme) for garnish

Instructions:

> Preheat the grill or oven.

> Thread chickpeas and vegetables onto skewers.

> Brush with olive oil and lemon marinade.

> Grill or bake until vegetables are tender and slightly charred.

> Garnish with fresh herbs before serving.

Health Benefits:

> Chickpeas provide protein and fiber.

> Vegetables offer vitamins and antioxidants.

Preparation Time: 25 minutes

8: Butternut Squash and Sage Risotto

Ingredients:

- 1 cup Arborio rice
- 1/2 cup dry white wine
- 4 cups vegetable broth, warmed
- 1 small butternut squash, diced
- 1 onion, finely chopped
- 2 cloves garlic, minced
- Fresh sage leaves
- Parmesan cheese (optional)
- Olive oil
- Salt and pepper to taste

Instructions:

- In a large pan, sauté onion and garlic in olive oil until translucent.
- Add Arborio rice and cook until lightly toasted.
- Pour in the white wine and cook until absorbed.
- Gradually add warm vegetable broth, stirring constantly.

- Add butternut squash and continue stirring until rice is creamy.
- Stir in fresh sage leaves, salt, and pepper.
- Optional: Garnish with Parmesan cheese before serving.

Health Benefits:

- Butternut squash provides vitamins and fiber.
- Arborio rice offers a source of energy.

Preparation Time: 40 minutes

9: Spaghetti Squash with Turkey Bolognese

Ingredients:

- 1 spaghetti squash, halved and seeds removed
- 1 lb ground turkey
- 1 onion, diced
- 2 cloves garlic, minced
- 1 can (15 oz) crushed tomatoes
- 1 teaspoon Italian seasoning
- Fresh basil for garnish
- Olive oil
- Salt and pepper to taste

Instructions:

- ➢ Preheat the oven to 400°F (200°C).
- ➢ Drizzle olive oil on spaghetti squash halves and season with salt and pepper.
- ➢ Place squash on a baking sheet, cut side down, and roast for 30-40 minutes.
- ➢ In a skillet, cook ground turkey until browned. Add onion and garlic.
- ➢ Pour in crushed tomatoes and Italian seasoning. Simmer until heated through.
- ➢ Scrape the spaghetti squash with a fork to create "noodles."
- ➢ Top with turkey Bolognese and garnish with fresh basil.

Health Benefits:

- ➢ Spaghetti squash offers a low-carb alternative to pasta.
- ➢ Turkey provides lean protein.

Preparation Time: 50 minutes

10: Vegan Chickpea and Spinach Curry

Ingredients:

- ➢ 1 can (15 oz) chickpeas, drained and rinsed
- ➢ 2 cups fresh spinach
- ➢ 1 onion, finely chopped
- ➢ 2 tomatoes, diced
- ➢ 1 can (15 oz) coconut milk
- ➢ 2 tablespoons curry powder
- ➢ 1 teaspoon turmeric
- ➢ 2 tablespoons vegetable oil
- ➢ Basmati rice for serving

Instructions:

- ➢ In a pan, sauté onion in vegetable oil until translucent.
- ➢ Add chickpeas, spinach, tomatoes, curry powder, and turmeric.
- ➢ Pour in coconut milk and simmer until spinach is wilted.
- ➢ Serve over basmati rice.

Health Benefits:

> Chickpeas provide protein and fiber.

> Spinach offers vitamins and antioxidants.

Preparation Time: 30 minutes

Snacks Recipes for Arthritis

1. Turmeric Roasted Chickpeas:

Ingredients:

> 1 can (15 oz) chickpeas, drained and rinsed

> 1 tablespoon olive oil

> 1 teaspoon turmeric

> 1/2 teaspoon cumin

> 1/2 teaspoon paprika

> Salt to taste

Instructions:

> Preheat the oven to 400°F (200°C).

> In a bowl, toss chickpeas with olive oil, turmeric, cumin, paprika, and salt.

> Spread chickpeas on a baking sheet in a single layer.

> Bake for 25-30 minutes, or until crispy, shaking the pan occasionally.

➢ Allow to cool before serving.

Health Benefits:

➢ Turmeric has anti-inflammatory properties that may help manage arthritis symptoms.

➢ Chickpeas are a good source of protein and fiber.

Preparation Time: 35 minutes

2. Spinach and Artichoke Dip:

Ingredients:

➢ 1 cup chopped spinach (fresh or frozen)

➢ 1 can (14 oz) artichoke hearts, drained and chopped

➢ 1 cup Greek yogurt

➢ 1/2 cup grated Parmesan cheese

➢ 1/2 cup light mayonnaise

➢ 1 clove garlic, minced

➢ Salt and pepper to taste

Instructions:

➢ Preheat oven to 375°F (190°C).

➢ In a bowl, mix together spinach, artichokes, Greek yogurt, Parmesan, mayonnaise, garlic, salt, and pepper.

➢ Transfer the mixture to a baking dish.

➢ Bake for 20-25 minutes or until bubbly and lightly browned.

➢ Serve with raw veggies or whole-grain crackers.

Health Benefits:

➢ Spinach and artichokes provide essential vitamins and antioxidants.

➢ Greek yogurt adds protein without excessive fat.

Preparation Time: 30 minutes

3. Quinoa Salad with Avocado and Walnuts:

Ingredients:

➢ 1 cup cooked quinoa

➢ 1 ripe avocado, diced

➢ 1/2 cup chopped walnuts

➢ 1/4 cup chopped fresh cilantro

➢ 1 tablespoon olive oil

➢ 1 tablespoon lemon juice

➢ Salt and pepper to taste

Instructions:

> In a bowl, combine cooked quinoa, diced avocado, walnuts, and cilantro.
> In a small bowl, whisk together olive oil, lemon juice, salt, and pepper.
> Drizzle the dressing over the quinoa mixture and toss gently.
> Chill in the refrigerator before serving.

Health Benefits:

> Quinoa is a whole grain rich in protein and fiber.
> Avocado provides healthy fats, and walnuts offer omega-3 fatty acids.

Preparation Time: 15 minutes

4. Baked Sweet Potato Chips:

Ingredients:

> 2 medium sweet potatoes, thinly sliced
> 2 tablespoons olive oil
> 1 teaspoon smoked paprika
> 1/2 teaspoon garlic powder
> Salt to taste

Instructions:

> Preheat oven to 375°F (190°C).
> In a bowl, toss sweet potato slices with olive oil, smoked paprika, garlic powder, and salt.
> Arrange the slices on a baking sheet in a single layer.
> Bake for 20-25 minutes or until crisp, flipping them halfway through.

Health Benefits:

> Sweet potatoes are rich in antioxidants and anti-inflammatory nutrients.
> Olive oil contains heart-healthy monounsaturated fats.

Preparation Time: 30 minutes

5. Berry and Chia Seed Pudding:

Ingredients:

> 1 cup mixed berries (strawberries, blueberries, raspberries)
> 2 tablespoons chia seeds
> 1 cup almond milk (or any preferred milk)
> 1 tablespoon honey or maple syrup

- ➤ 1/2 teaspoon vanilla extract

Instructions:

- ➤ In a jar or bowl, mix chia seeds, almond milk, honey (or maple syrup), and vanilla extract.
- ➤ Stir well and refrigerate for at least 2 hours or overnight.
- ➤ Before serving, layer the chia pudding with mixed berries.

Health Benefits:

- ➤ Chia seeds are rich in omega-3 fatty acids and fiber.
- ➤ Berries provide antioxidants and vitamins.

Preparation Time: 2 hours (including chilling time)

6. Roasted Red Pepper Hummus:

Ingredients:

- ➤ 1 can (15 oz) chickpeas, drained and rinsed
- ➤ 1/3 cup tahini
- ➤ 1/4 cup lemon juice
- ➤ 1/4 cup roasted red peppers (from a jar)
- ➤ 2 cloves garlic, minced
- ➤ 2 tablespoons olive oil

> Salt and cumin to taste

Instructions:

> In a food processor, blend chickpeas, tahini, lemon juice, roasted red peppers, garlic, olive oil, salt, and cumin until smooth.
> Adjust seasoning to taste.
> Serve with sliced veggies or whole-grain pita.

Health Benefits:

> Chickpeas provide protein and fiber.
> Olive oil offers healthy monounsaturated fats.

Preparation Time: 15 minutes

7. Cucumber and Greek Yogurt Dip:

Ingredients:

> 1 cucumber, finely diced
> 1 cup Greek yogurt
> 1 clove garlic, minced
> 1 tablespoon fresh dill, chopped
> 1 tablespoon lemon juice
> Salt and pepper to taste

Instructions:

- In a bowl, combine cucumber, Greek yogurt, garlic, dill, lemon juice, salt, and pepper.
- Mix well and refrigerate for at least 30 minutes before serving.
- Serve with cucumber slices or whole-grain crackers.

Health Benefits:

- Greek yogurt adds protein and probiotics.
- Cucumber provides hydration and vitamins.

Preparation Time: 10 minutes

8. Almond and Apricot Energy Balls:

Ingredients:

- 1 cup almonds, finely chopped
- 1 cup dried apricots, chopped
- 1/2 cup rolled oats
- 2 tablespoons honey
- 1 teaspoon vanilla extract
- 1/2 teaspoon ground cinnamon
- Shredded coconut for coating (optional)

Instructions:

> In a food processor, combine almonds, dried apricots, rolled oats, honey, vanilla extract, and cinnamon.
> Pulse until the mixture comes together.
> Roll the mixture into small balls and coat with shredded coconut if desired.
> Refrigerate for at least 30 minutes before serving.

Health Benefits:

> Almonds provide healthy fats and vitamin E.
> Apricots offer fiber and natural sweetness.

Preparation Time: 20 minutes

9. Salmon and Avocado Nori Rolls:

Ingredients:

> 4 sheets nori seaweed
> 1/2 cup cooked quinoa
> 1/2 cup cooked and flaked salmon
> 1 avocado, sliced
> 1/2 cucumber, julienned
> Soy sauce for dipping (low-sodium)

Instructions:

- ➢ Place a sheet of nori on a bamboo sushi mat.
- ➢ Spread a thin layer of quinoa on the nori, leaving a small border at the top.
- ➢ Arrange salmon, avocado, and cucumber along the bottom edge.
- ➢ Roll tightly and seal the edge with a bit of water.
- ➢ Slice into bite-sized pieces and serve with soy sauce.

Health Benefits:

- ➢ Salmon provides omega-3 fatty acids.
- ➢ Avocado adds healthy fats and creaminess.

Preparation Time: 25 minutes

10. Greek Salad Skewers:

Ingredients:

- ➢ Cherry tomatoes
- ➢ Cucumber, cut into chunks
- ➢ Feta cheese, cubed
- ➢ Kalamata olives
- ➢ Extra virgin olive oil
- ➢ Fresh oregano, chopped

> Balsamic glaze for drizzling

Instructions:

> Thread cherry tomatoes, cucumber chunks, feta cheese cubes, and olives onto skewers.
> Drizzle with olive oil and sprinkle with chopped oregano.
> Serve with a side of balsamic glaze for dipping.

Health Benefits:

> Tomatoes provide antioxidants, and cucumber adds hydration.
> Feta cheese offers calcium and protein.

Preparation Time: 15 minutes

CONCLUSION

Embracing an arthritis-friendly diet doesn't mean sacrificing flavor or enjoyment.

By incorporating nutrient-rich ingredients with anti-inflammatory properties, these recipes not only cater to those seeking relief from arthritis symptoms but also offer a delicious way to maintain overall well-being.

From the vibrant Turmeric Roasted Chickpeas to the refreshing Greek Salad Skewers, each dish is a testament to the power of wholesome, thoughtfully selected ingredients. Remember, making informed dietary choices can be a valuable ally in the journey towards managing arthritis and promoting a healthier, more vibrant life.

So, dive into these recipes, savor the goodness, and discover how a thoughtful approach to nutrition can make a meaningful difference in your day-to-day well-being.

Here's to enjoying delicious, nourishing meals that contribute to your health and vitality!